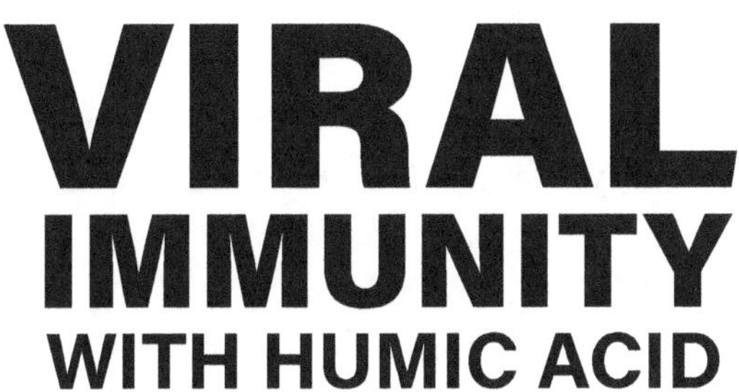

VIRAL IMMUNITY
WITH HUMIC ACID

Dr. Howard Peiper

VIRAL IMMUNITY
WITH HUMIC ACID

NEW UPDATED EDITION

Table of Contents

Part One:

The Virus at Our Doorstep 5
So, What Is a Virus? 6
Welcome to the Viral Realm - 4,000 Types of Viruses 7
Types of Viral Infections 10
Viruses: Common and Exotic - A review of the Key
 Viral Agents in Humans 11
Viruses That Affect Animals 17

Part Two:

Unlocking Mother Earth's Chamber of Secrets 20

Part Three:

Clinical Studies 25
Protocol for Taking Humic Acid 29
Frequently Asked Questions 30
Testimonials 33
 Viral Treatment of Humans 32
 Viral Treatment of Animals 34

Resources Directory 36

About the Author 37

Author's Statement

A very real threat from emerging viruses does exist and must be taken with the utmost seriousness. The possibility that the world could be thrown into a crisis of unprecedented proportions is real. The main question is not if we will have a viral epidemic, rather is is what direction is the current epidemic of microbial illnesses taking.

Howard Peiper, N.D.

Part One

The Virus at our Doorstep

Viruses recognize no international borders or time zones. They have no obligations to country, race, social status, or gender. Rich and poor, alike, are victims of viral infections which, if given the opportunity, may travel over extraordinarily long distances. In 1983, the Asian tiger mosquito (the mosquito that transmits dengue fever virus) was found for the first time in the United States. The mosquito larvae were transported on a cargo ship from Southeast Asia as stowaways in accumulated rainwater inside automobile tires.

In our modern world, viruses and other infectious microbes can easily hitch rides on international flights to and from any major city. A tourist visiting Thailand can bring home a strain of human immunodeficiency virus from a sexual encounter in Bangkok. A grandmother visiting her family in San Francisco following a stay in China can harbor a potent influenza virus in her lungs and pass it to her grand children who transmit it to other children in preschool.

We know viruses have been with us a long time. Archaeological evidence indicates smallpox developed along with civilization in the river basin agricultural settlements of Asia and the Middle East as early as 10,000 years ago. We also know that most viral epidemic diseases were unheard of in the New World before the arrival of early settlers. Viruses are not only the cause of many infectious diseases, ranging from the common cold to slow death of AIDS and the frightening fevers, but they have dramatically influenced history as well.

Viruses have toppled dynasties, changed the outcomes of wars, and altered populations. In the twentieth century, smallpox alone killed and estimated 300 million people. In the sixteenth and seventeenth centuries small pox killed the emperors of Japan and Burma as well as many Kings and queens of Europe. The 1918-19 epidemic of Spanish influenza killed 33 million people in less than a year. Causing more deaths than all the massive military casualties of World War I.

Viruses not only infect humans but all living things including plants, animals, bird and sea creatures. In 1999, seal plague virus killed 3,600 seals in the United Kingdom. Canine distemper and other common animal viruses kill our pets as well as livestock. Rinderpest, or cattle plague, killed an estimated 3 million cattle annually in South Africa during the 1930s. Viruses are everywhere, and due to their microscopic size they also infect the invisible world, including bacteria, fungi, and protozoa.

So, What is a Virus?

Viruses are very small. Viruses are referred to as subcellular organisms, meaning they are smaller than cells, smaller than bacteria, and certainly smaller than most human host cells. Viruses are so minute they can maintain their ability to infect even after passing through filters small enough to strain out all bacteria. In fact, they are so small that they can only be seen by the most powerful of electron microscopes.

Viruses are Parasites. Viruses are intracellular molecular parasites. They enter the body silently and, as in the cases of HIV and hepatitis C viruses, they often do so without notice. Using our cells to manufacture substances needed for their own replication and life cycle. They have no metabolic life of their own outside a host cell, which makes them depended on living cells for their existence. Viruses have a receptor binging protein that allows them to attach to other cells and convert them to virus-producing mini-factories. They do not make their own energy or proteins for survival and cannot reproduce without the assistance of cellular material from other living cells. Viruses grow and multiply only within other living cells - human, animal, plan or bacteria. Outside the host cell, a virus is not alive and exists in a world between the living and nonliving.

Viruses are genetically lean. The basic viral particle or individual virus is called a virion. It consists of a nucleic acid genome in which the viruses hereditary information is stored, surrounded by a shell of protein. Unlike most living cells, viruses do not have cell walls composed of a plasma membrane. Instead, a protein coat called a capsid (which may also contain lipids and sugars), protect the viral genome.

All living cells contain two types of genetic material, RNA and DNA, but viruses possess only one type, either RNA or DNA. They also have a very small number of genes compared or other cells. For comparison, the human immunodeficiency virus (HIV) has fewer than ten genes; a larger virus like smallpox contains around 300 genes, but even the smallest bacteria contains around 7500 genes, and a human cell has over 90,000 genes.

Welcome to the Viral Realm - 4,000 Types of Viruses

There are 4,000 known types of viruses, with new viruses being discovered regularly, but less than three percent of those known viruses are well characterized. Indeed, at least sixty have been identified since 1986. Classification of viruses is based on several criteria, mainly by the type of nucleic acid (DNA or RNA) and by whether the genome contains a single strand (ss) or double strand (ds) of genetic material. For example, smallpox is a dsDNA virus and HIV has an ssRNA genome.

Among the DNA types are viruses that cause:

- *chicken pox*
- *herpes simplex*
- *smallpox*
- *shingles*
- *warts*
- *hepatitis B*
- *common cold*

Among the RNA types are viruses that cause:

- *yellow fever*
- *bronchitis*
- *rubella*
- *corona*
- *measles*
- *hepatitis C*
- *encephalitis*
- *polio*
- *influenza*
- *HIV*

Viral carriers and natural hosts.

To understand how viruses cause disease, it is important for us to define some commonly used terms. Although the specific origin of viruses is unknown, it is an accepted theory that they usually descend from a parent source already existing in nature and then spread from animal to animal and then from animals to humans. The infected bacterium/plant/animal/person is referred to as the host.

Although the individual person is understandably concerned only with his/her own ailment, what many people are unaware of is that even the most common of viral diseases originates in animal hosts. For example, though influenza virus causes common respiratory infections worldwide, most strains of it originate in China where the natural hosts are livestock, especially pigs, chickens and ducks.

Other animal hosts that carry viruses infecting humans are:

- migratory waterfowl
- birds
- rodents
- monkeys

Humans can also carry viral disease, and certainly human groups are more likely to carry viruses than those who are isolated from others. Interestingly, children are the most common hosts and carriers for many viruses such as the common cold and measles. Due to their high exposure to sickness, healthcare workers are also frequent carriers for viruses. The most seriously affected, and the groups in which the most mortality are seen are the very young and very old. This is why public health measures concentrate on vaccinations for children and flu shots for seniors. Since healthcare workers, like doctors and nurses, are particularly at risk due to their daily exposure to sick people, hey are also encouraged to be vaccinated against influenza virus.

Viruses have a unique way of promoting their own life cycle. First they infect the host, often causing sickness in the process. Then they pass out of the host, usually in body fluids. For example, rotaviruses that cause traveler's diarrhea (a serious and even lethal illness) pass from the body of the host to the feces. In every gram of infected feces reside about one billion rotaviruses. If sanitation measures are not in place, these active viruses readily enter the water or food supply to infect others.

Influenza is spread by people expelling the virus-laden particles of saliva and mucus by coughing and sneezing. Every person in the immediate vicinity then inhales these particles.

How Viruses Enter the Body.
Viruses typically enter the human body through one of three locations: the respiratory tract (nose, throat, and lungs); the *gastrointestinal tract* (mouth, stomach, and intestines); and the *genitourinary tract* (the sex organs and urinary area).

Viruses gain entry into the body through the respiratory tract when their victims *inhale* air into which people with that virus have coughed or sneezed. Viruses of the gastrointestinal tract generally enter the body in *food contaminated* in preparation, as is the case with hepatitis A. *Sexual intercourse* is the prime access for certain viruses, such as HIV and herpes, through the genitourinary tract.   Viruses also have been quick to exploit modern medical practices. The normal portals of entry now include: direct blood-to-blood transmission, such as in blood transfusions (although unintentional, blood transfusions greatly contributed to the spread of HIV and hepatitis B and C); and by shared hypodermic needle use which has caused wide spread viral transmission of hepatitis C among intravenous drug users.

In effect, the immune system receives a surprise attack and its response must be appropriately strong enough to eliminate the virus. Often, as in HIV and HCV, there is no immediate immune response, as the virus has stealth mechanisms to outsmart the body's natural defenses. Only after the virus is well established in the liver or nervous system does the immune system react, and even then it may be in a manner that is more destructive to the host than to the virus. Some viruses like German measles and HIV can spread from mother to child, passing through the placenta during pregnancy. In the case of herpes simplex virus, a baby can be infected from the mother's blood when passing through the birth canal. Some viruses such as cytomegalovirus (CMV) and HIV can also be passed along in breast milk.

Types of Viral Infections

The list of diseases caused by viruses is immense and ranges from the common cold to cancer. Viruses not only cause specific diseases with clear diagnostic symptoms, but can also cause a constellation of symptoms that can defy diagnosis. Some viral diseases mimic other illnesses (for example, fatigue caused by anemia), or secondary inflammation (joint pain associated with arthritis). Certain viruses have specific affinity for only one type of tissue such as the liver or skin, while others an attraction to the body organs and systems. Viruses can cause localized infections such as warts or a sore throat, or a generalized infection such as in influenza, in which your whole body feels sick.

The Virus and Cancer Connection.
Cancer remains one of the leading causes of death in the developed countries. One out of every three (and it is rapidly approaching one out of two) individuals will develop some form of cancer. Oncogenesis, the term used to describe the development of cancer, has long been associated with viruses. Since viruses are so small and can also directly interact with genetic material, viruses can potentially gain access to any site and cell in the body. It is therefore no surprise that they can also cause cancer. Among the more widespread of the virally induced cancers is cervical cancer. Cervical cancer is one of the most common cancers in women, caused by the papillomavirus, a member of the same viral family that causes warts. Other forms of cancer from viruses are: hepatocellular carcinoma caused by hepatitis B and C; and, Kaposi's sarcoma, caused by a newly discovered herpes virus, HHV-8, which occurs in AIDS.

A New Viral Plague?
Historically, it appears diseases go into latent or dormant phases and reemerge when conditions are favorable for their proliferation, just as they do in our bodies. What is of concern now is not only the increasing variety of new viruses and other infectious diseases, but the weakening of our natural immunity from toxic pollutants and stress allowing the

spread of potent viruses into areas of dense human population. Every element is in place for a new plague.

In the past, when population density was considerably smaller and the balanced laws of nature still ruled the plains, savannas, forests, and mountains, human viral diseases were rare and appeared primarily in the overcrowded and filthy cities. After the great smallpox epidemics that occurred during the clash of cultures when Europeans colonized the rest of the plant, viral diseases were relatively quiescent. The new viral diseases that have been recently described are a phenomenon of the late twentieth century, and they will be of great concern to us in the twenty-first century.

Viruses: Common and Exotic - A Review of the Key Viral Agents in Humans

To better understand the principles and methods of using a natural antiviral called humic acid effectively, it helps to have some knowledge about the key agents on the viral playing field. In this section, let's look at the most common and most important of the current viruses.

Among the viruses presented in this section, the one most likely to cause a pandemic (a worldwide epidemic) is the flu, perhaps already the most common and widely known of all viral diseases. Indeed, it is a real threat, and one that was a likelihood of occurring the next decade or so.

Coronaviruses
Coronaviruses make up a large family of viruses that can infect birds and mammals, including humans. These viruses have been responsible for several outbreaks around the world, including the severe acute respiratory syndrome (SARS), the Middle East respiratory syndrome (MERS) and recently, a novel coronavirus (SARS-Cov-2), also known as COVID-19. While some coronaviruses have caused devastating epidemics, others cause mild to moderate respiratory infections, like the common cold.

Coronaviruses can be transmitted between humans through respiratory droplets that infected people expel when they breathe, cough or sneeze. The symptoms typically cause a respiratory infection with mild to severe flu-like conditions, however, the exact symptoms vary depending on the type of coronavirus.

The four common human coronaviruses can cause people to develop a runny nose, headache, cough, sore throat, difficulty breathing, body aches, chills, and fever. In individuals, including those with cardiopulmonary disease or a weakened immune system, the viral infection can progress to a more severe lower-respiratory infection such as pneumonia or bronchitis.

Dengue

Dengue (also called "break-bone fever") is another of the Old World diseases once common in North America. Today, it is mostly concentrated in Southeast Asia, where thousands of cases are reported annually. Dengue hemorrhagic fever shock syndrome (DHFS), a condition once found only in children, is now in the U.S., the Caribbean and South America. Worldwide, dengue infects between 60 and 90 million people each year and is considered the most common mosquito-borne virus.

Ebola

Next to AIDS, Ebola is one of the most terrifying viruses, as attested to in recent media coverage. There are three types of Ebola, which is also a bleeding fever like Hanta and dengue, but only two types affect humans. The third type infects monkeys, and is epidemic in parts of Africa, but Ebola has "cousins" that occur in other parts of the world including Europe, South America and Asia.

Hepatitis

Hepatitis, a general medical term for liver inflammation, is not caused by only one virus. Through many different viruses cause infections in the liver, including Epstein-Barr virus, three main viruses cause damage to human liver cells. Hepatitis A (HAV) caused by an RNA virus and is contracted through feces containing viral particles which then contaminate water or food consumed by humans.

Hepatitis B (HBV), sometimes referred to as serum hepatitis, is a serious blood-borne viral illness that can lead to chronic liver disease, liver cancer, or if its course is severe, rapid infection, can cause death. It is transmitted in blood and other body fluids, like semen and breast milk.

Hepatitis B (HCV) is considered a blood-borne virus, however it now appears there are modes of transmission other than directly through the blood. Known sources of infection include: 1) injection drug use; 2) needle-stick accidents by health worker; 3) contact with infected blood product; 4) sexual contact with menstrual blood infected persons; 5) infants born to infected women; 6) tattoos; and, 7) shared toothbrushes and razors.

Herpes Virus

Herpes viruses cause a variety of infections in humans, including cold sores (canker sores), sexually transmitted infections, and neurological diseases. They are also implicated in certain forms of cancer logical diseases. They are also implicated in certain forms of cancer and chronic disease states like chronic fatigue immune deficiency syndrome (CFIDS). What makes herpes viruses such a potential problem is that 95 percent of the world's population harbors some form of herpes virus, and after initial exposure and primary infection, all of these viruses enter a dormant state within different tissue cells, such as skin or cells of the nervous system. Infection is therefore permanent and latency of the virus is life long.

HIV

Human immunodeficiency virus (HIV) may be nature's perfect virus. It spreads by an act common to almost all humans-sexual activity. The infection progresses slowly, allowing for a host carrier to spread to other individuals before full symptoms appear. Once in the body, it invades specific cells of the immune system causing increased vulnerability to a wide variety of fatal infections. The virus mutates rapidly, defying antiviral drugs and, when suppressed by drugs, it is capable of laying latent indefinitely.

Influenza

Influenza is called the "last of the great uncontrolled plagues," and some epidemiologists believe that we are imminently due for an influenza epidemic of plague proportions similar to that of 1918.

There are three known types of influenza that infect humans influenza A, B and C. The most important of these is influenza A, which has over thirty known subtypes. Influenza virus causes acute outbreaks of severe respiratory tract infection. It has a remarkable ability to evade individual host defenses and to undergo massive genetic changes that prevent human populations from acquiring any measure of permanent immunity against it.

Infection from the influenza virus is simple and extremely effective and universal. It occurs from breathing contaminated air containing viral particles spread by coughing and sneezing. After an incubation period of two to three days, symptoms start abruptly with shivering, malaise, fatigue, headache, and aching of the limbs and back.

Marburg

Marburg virus is a re-emerging pathogen that poses a significant threat to human health. This naturally occurring virus can cause a fulminating hemorrhagic disease with a severe shock syndrome and high mortality in both humans and nonhuman primates – also known as Marburg hemorrhagic fever.

Marburg hemorrhagic fever is characterized by an abrupt onset presenting with fever, chills, and myalgia. Two features of the disease are critical in its pathogenesis: endothelial damage orchestrated by both the virus and the up-regulation of toxic cytokines (with extensive vascular leakage therefore) and disseminated intravascular coagulation which leads to serious thrombocytopenia.

As a result, severe hemorrhage can ensue at several body sites within approximately 5 to 7 days after the onset of symptoms. Bleeding from the nose, gums, and eyes is commonly observed, whereas considerable gastrointestinal hemorrhage will often manifest as frank blood in the stool or vomit. Dehydration is a frequent consequence.

Mosquito-, Tick- and Rodent-spread Viruses

The viruses in this group include a wide range of viral diseases from several different viral families. Insects spread most of these viruses, particularly the mosquito. Among them are well-known diseases such as yellow fever, dengue, Lyme disease, and newly emerging ones like Ebola and hanta viruses.

Viral Gastroenteritis

Viral gastroenteritis, also called "cruise-ship virus" or Norwalk/Norwalk-like virus. Symptoms appear suddenly after a very brief incubation period and include vomiting, nausea, diarrhea abdominal cramping, mild fever, and headache. Humans are the only source for these viruses. These viruses do not multiply outside the human body. The viruses are present in the feces of infected persons and can be transmitted to others when hands are not thoroughly washed following a bowl movement. When an infected person who did not wash after toileting handles food that is not later cooked, others who eat the food can become infected.

Warts

Human papilloma viruses (HPV) cause common warts, plantar warts, and genital warts. There are over 80 known different types of HPV, and though most are benign, some types can develop into cancer. The most important of the potentially malignant type are those that occur in the female cervix, especially HPV types 16 and 18. These may often be found by a physician performing routine pelvic examinations.

Yellow Fever and Other Viral Disasters

Diseases caused by "blood-sucking" insects produce an array of viral illnesses that range from mild flu-like symptoms to death. Of these the most severe is yellow fever, which is carried by the same mosquito as dengue. Yellow fever is a hemorrhagic disease that attacks the liver causing jaundice, necrosis (death of cells), and death. It is still common in tropical Africa, Latin America, and Asia.

A number of other insect-borne viruses that cause illnesses in America include ***West Nile Fever, California encephalitis,*** and ***Colorado tick fever.*** Most of these viruses cause (or can lead to) inflammation of the central nervous system. Rodents, such as squirrels, mice, and rats, spread viruses in their droppings when they forage for food. The contaminated food is then eaten, or dried fecal matter contaminates the air is subsequently inhaled. The most notorious of rodent-related viruses in hanta. In 1993, an emerging Hantavirus was identified in New Mexico. It attacks the kidneys and can cause lunch inflammation, internal bleeding, and death. Lyme disease is another serious illness caused by a virus transmitted by the deer tick.

Zika

The Zika virus is a mosquito-borne viral infection that primarily occurs in tropical and subtropical areas of the world. Most people infected with the Zika virus have no signs and symptoms, while others report mild fever, rash and muscle pain. Other signs and symptoms may include headache, red eyes (conjunctivitis) and a general feeling of discomfort. Zika virus is also called Zika or Zika virus disease.

Zika virus infections during pregnancy have been linked to miscarriage and can cause microcephaly, a potentially fatal congenital brain condition. The Zika virus also may cause other neurological disorders such as Guillain-Barre syndrome.

As many as 4 out of 5 people infected with the Zika virus have no signs or symptoms. When symptoms do occur, they usually begin two to seven days after a person is bitten by an infected mosquito. Signs and symptoms of the Zika virus most commonly include: mild fever, rash, joint or muscle ache, rash, headache, and/or red eye (conjunctivitis).

Viruses That Affect Animals

Dogs

Canine parvovirus, also called parvoviral enteritis, is a contagious disease of dogs that affects puppies more often than older dogs. The disease was uncommon before the summer of 1978, when it became an epidemic in the United States. The fatality rate is extremely high. Canine parvovirus infects the entire intestinal tract of a dog, causing diarrhea, vomiting, dehydration, and malaise. Puppies usually develop a high fever, but older dogs may have subnormal temperatures. Some dogs also develop a cough or swelling of the cornea of the eye. The illness usually begins suddenly, and without treatment the animal often dies within a few days.

Distemper is a highly contagious disease of dogs, wolves, coyotes and ferrets. It is caused by a virus that is easily spread through the air and by contaminated objects, much like the cold virus spreads in people. Though the disease occurs more often in young dogs, hose of any age may contract distemper. This is especially true of animals under stress or those that are relatively isolated from other dogs. Signs range from those of a mild respiratory problem, such as runny eyes and nose, to severe diarrhea, vomiting and seizures. Many recovered dogs are left with uncontrollable muscle or limb jerking and/ or periodic convulsions.

Other viruses that affect dogs:

- Parainfluenza
- Hepatitis
- Leptospirosis

Cats

One of the most dangerous infectious diseases of cats today is caused by the feline leukemia virus (FeLV). FeLV is a retrovirus that is specific to cats only and is the most common cause of serious illness and death in domestic cats. It suppresses the immune system, impairing the cat's ability to fight infections. It may also cause anemia, leukemia and some forms of cancer. FeLV cannot be transmitted to humans (including children) or other species such as dogs.

Feline immunodeficiency virus (FIV), is a widespread viral infection that attacks the immune system of cats. It is often referred to as "feline AIDS." The virus ravages a cat's immune system, stopping it from effectively combating other diseases and infections. Infected cats eventually fall prey to a wide variety of secondary illnesses that overwhelmingly prove fatal. FIV is not transmissible to people or dogs.

Other viruses that affect cats:

- coronavirus
- respiratory disease complex
- cat flu (Feline Respiratory Viruses {FCV})
- Feline Infectious Enteritis (FIE)

Horses

Most viral diseases tend to spread with great rapidity through the herd with all susceptible animals becoming infected in a short time. With some viral diseases the carrier state is quite common. As a general rule, viral infections are characterized by sudden onset fever, depressed white blood cell count, absence of pus formation, and lack of specific response to drug therapy.

A number of viruses affect the equine respiratory tract. They are influenza, herpes, rhinopneumonitis (EVR), reo, and arteritis viruses. Adenovirus pneumonia has also been reported in association with combined immunodeficiency in Arabian foals. Equine herpesvirus type 4 (EHV-4, rhinopneumonitis) and influenza are commonly involved in clinical infections. Equine herpesvirus type 1 (EHV-1) is primarily associated with abortion but is recognized as an occasional cause of respiratory disease. Vaccines do not always prevent infection.

Several viruses are capable of causing encephalitis in horses. These are classified as arboviruses. Arboviruses are viruses that are transmitted by mosquitoes. Occurrence of arboviruses is sporadic and seasonal. Where the disease is endemic, outbreaks can be anticipated a week or two following peak mosquito season. West Nile virus falls into the arbovirus classification. The virus multiplies in the horse's blood system, crosses the blood brain barrier, and infects the brain. The virus interferes with normal central nervous system functioning and causes inflammation of the brain.

Other viruses that affect horses:

- Strangle (distemper or shipping fever)
- Vesicular stomatitis
- Equine influenza
- Equine Virus Abortion

Part II

Unlocking Mother Earth's Chamber of Secrets

Humates

Sealed away from wind and rain for millions of years are great deposits of animal and plant materials that have decomposed and then compressed together by the millions of tons of earth over them. This process locks in their nutrients providing seventy-two natural ingredients.

Humate is a safe material existing in all soils. It has been around since the beginning of time. The romans were aware of the benefits of Humates, but it was not until the 18th century that scientists discovered humic acid (see note below), and not until the early 1960s was science able to find a way to analyze it to determine its humic acid content. Today, scientists have discovered a missing link in our food chain, and they have drawn the conclusion that rapidly increasing degenerative diseases worldwide may be directly related to the absence of humic acid in the human diet.

Humic acid is a long chain molecule, which is dark brown, high in molecular weight, and is soluble in an alkali solution. It is the part of the soil responsible for composting and transferring the nutrients from the earth to the living organism. Humic acid material accompanies the nutrient into the organism and performs many benefits.

Nutritional experts now know that in addition to vitamins and minerals, humic acid is a third and vitally important nutrient required for health. These breakthrough discoveries are supported by little published and even secret medical research coming from top institutions around the world, medical schools, hospitals, clinics and pharmaceutical labs.

The reasons most of the world has not yet been informed about this medical discovery are complicated. Many research medical institutions are in the business of making enormous profits from developing synthetic, patented drugs, and they would prefer that you not know about natural solutions. Pharmaceutical companies have been rushing to patent synthetic versions of humic acid (a natural substance) with dozens of patents currently being approved. They will never be able to match Mother Nature's handiwork, however, because this substance is far too complex. An estimated 80 percent of pharmaceutical drugs are tiny, isolated, synthetic fractions and cannot even come close to this *whole* and *complete* "missing line" from Mother Nature.

What exactly is this miraculous substance?

Humic acid. Scientists have most appropriately referred to it as the antiviral answer. One of the many reasons for excitement involves the effects humic acid exhibits when dissolved in water (or combined with body fluids). Humic acid is the smallest, most complex, most highly refined naturally occurring water-soluble substance on Earth. tiny amounts remarkably transform the molecular structure of water, making it intensely more active and penetrable. Humic acid then assists water in its job of dissolving and transporting. It helps carry nutrients into the cell and waste products away from the cell, while also assisting in neutralizing toxins and invaders.

Humic acid has the dramatic ability to penetrate even deadly ultramicroscopic viruses.

As we have previously discussed, viruses are super small and live only deep inside the cells of plants, animals and humans. Viruses even live inside other microscopic disease causing organisms, where they "hitch a ride." Viruses encapsulate themselves in an impenetrable protein barrier where defense mechanisms cannot reach them. Humic acid puts a coating around the viruses and preventing the virus from adhering to a healthy cell. The viruses then become vulnerable to attack by the immune system. Yet this is only the beginning. Humic acid also has the amazing ability to alert the immune system to the virus or disease invader and to regulate and strengthen the immune system!

Scientists have determined that to successfully treat many serious diseases, including those caused by viruses, the immune system needs to be controlled selectively. Humic acid is able to do this naturally by suppressing certain immune responses while increasing others.

Humic acid's ability to selectively inhibit/complement the body's immune response is one of the reasons it has been successful in treating and even curing diseases traditionally thought to be incurable.

Historically, as documented in the Chinese Materia Medica pharmacological compendium dating back to the 15th century, a then famous medical doctor, Li Shi Zhen, used humic acid as the active ingredient in the treatment of infectious ulcerous growth and female hemorrhage disease. These treatises showed humic acid to be an efficient anti-inflammatory and flood-coagulating agent.

More recently, many reports on the beneficial use of humic acid for human health and medicine have been published. Many medical schools and hospitals in China have engaged in extensive studies on the toxicology and pathological aspects of humic acid and their clinical applications. Hundreds of research papers have now been published nationally in China, while many have appeared in international journals and have been presented at conferences outside of China. Chinese doctors now use humic related medicines to reduce inflammation, increase circulation, control bleeding, to regulate the immune and hormone systems, to heal digestive tract disorders, and as an anticancer and anti-tumor therapy. Research shows that humic acid naturally acts as a massive broad-spectrum antibiotic and antiviral medication equal to or even superior to those known and produced by the pharmaceutical industry today.

Clinical studies show that negative side effects are non-existent when using humic acid at the recommended dosage. No problems or negative side effects have ever been reported by an in the scientific literature. Extensive laboratory and clinical testing has proven absolute safety for human internal and external use.

What enhances humic acid's effectiveness?

Humates contain both humic and fulvic acids. Fulvic acids is a chelator and "carries" the minerals. Humic acid is the dilator, increasing the cell wall permeability. The increased permeability facilitated by the humic acid allows easier transfer of the minerals from the blood to the bones and cells. Humic acid also encapsulates the viruses in our body, thus making the viruses vulnerable to attack by the immune system. It further prevents the viruses from reproducing. The agents for this are called *viral fusion inhibitors* (through a special proprietary process, the humic acid is specially treated and sterilized). This process makes this particular humic acid the most effective antiviral product on the market.

Benefits obtained from a consistent long-term plan of dietary supplementation and topical use of humic acid include:

- provides increased resistance to cold and flu, infection and disease;
- cleanses, neutralizes and removes toxins;
- supercharges our immune system;
- assists in purging parasites, pathogens and viruses from your body
- creates a feeling of well being immediately;
- restores your body to is optimum potential over time.

Other Antiviral Remedies

Homeopathic preparations are the world's second most popular form of medicine. The approach of homeopathy is to trigger the body's defense system with small doses of the substances that stimulate healing in the body. Homeopathic preparations use the smallest possible dosage to produce the desired response. This results in remedies that are highly effective remarkably safe, and do not produce unwanted side effects.

Several studies and clinical trials examining the efficacy for the treatment of influenza of two homeopathic preparations reported remarkable findings. Anas Barbariae and Influenzinum were studied and tested. Recent double-blind, randomized, and placebo controlled clinical trails published in the peer-reviewed British Journal of Clinical Pharmacology and British Homeopathic Journal showed that Anas Barbariae provided a statistically significant action in decreasing flu-like symptoms, including cough, runny nose, sore throat, and muscle pain, as well as shortening the duration of the disease. In a documented 9-year study using Influenzinum as a preventative, 9 out of 10 participants were free of flu symptoms.

In the homeopathic *materia medica*, dozens of remedies are listed for use in viral conditions, and since classical homeopathic prescribing focuses on the constitution of the patient and not the pathology of the disease, the repertory of possible remedies is immense.

Special homeopathic substances that are used as a antiviral remedy:

- Anas Barbariae Hepatis et Cordis Extractum - For relief of all flu symptoms
- Eupatorium Perfoliatum - For relief of vomiting, coughing, sneezing, headache, and aching/soreness in back of limbs
- Gelsemium - For relief of chills, dizziness, drowsiness, sneezing, heavy feeling, dull headache, dry cough, heavy chest and vertigo
- Influenzinum A, B, C - Specifically for all flu symptoms
- Kreosotum - For relief of feverish sensation over the whole body, shivering, chills, coughs, phlegm and copious expectoration
- Tuberculinum Aviare - Acts on lungs, bronchia, tickling, and irritating coughs
- Tuberculinum - For fever with profuse seating, chilling in all stages of fever, dry hard cough, yellow or green sputum and pneumonia after the flu
- Veratrum Viride - For relief of high fever in evening

Part III

Clinical Studies

"Medical studies show that difficult respiratory illnesses common in children are readily resolved with humic acid dietary supplementation. Humic acid is found in rich organic soil and also certain ancient plant deposits. Humic acid has the power to protect against cancer and the related cancer-causing viruses. Studies often show reversal of deadly cancers and tumors using special humic substance therapies."

R. Klocking and M. Sprossing: Experientia,
1972 28(5) pp. 607-608

Human Case Study Data on AIDS

Nigeria, Africa - April, 2003
- three males, 20-30 years old African decent HIV+
- one tablet four times a day
- viral load went from 15,000-18,000 to undetectable within 60 days

Taiwan - June, 2003
- two males and one female 30-40 years old Chinese decent HIV+
- one tablet four times a day
- viral load went from 16,000-20,000 to undetectable within 60 days

United States - June, 2003
- two males and one female 20-40 years old Caucasian HIV+
- one tablet three times a day
  one patient reported to be in advanced stages of AIDS
- viral load went from 12,000-15,000 to undetectable within 18-30 days

Broad Spectrum Antiviral Effectiveness of Humates
National Institutes of Health (NIH) - August, 2002

This report presents the results of toxicology, cell proliferation and efficacy-testing work carried out on humic acid. Antiviral properties were examined on: viral gastroenteritis (cruise-ship virus), herpes, influenza, chicken pox/shingles, mononucleosis, and hemorrhagic fevers (Ebola and Hanta). Standard toxicity tests were run on humic acid used in the tests. Humic acid was found to bind to cell surfaces and was in no way toxic to the cell. Testing was done to see if any effect was observed on normal cell growth of healthy tissues. Observations from the tests indicated no ill effect on the cell growth or reproduction.

Conclusion: Humic acids exhibit effects, both as a preventive and a curative, for a broad range of viruses. Testing also indicated that humic acid taken before introduction of the virus exhibited a strong prophylactic effect.

Experimental starting points and prospects of using humic acids in medicine
Biological Sciences: Dr. T.C. Lotosh, Moscow, Russia - October, 1991

"The analysis of action of physiologically active humic acid is given. Using pharmaco-biological tests and modeling of the diseases, a high anti-toxic effect of humic acid and possibility to use it in medicine and veterinary sciences as non-specific pharmacy raising the organism resistance to the action of different unfavorable factors is proved.

"Scientists revealed humic acid harmless with respect to blood, cardi-vascular system, endocrine system and other vitally important organs using patho-histological and histochemical methods. Humic acid does not cause any allergic reaction, anaphylaxis to other medicines."

"A special study of the influence of humic acid on the antitoxin of the liver was researched. The fact that the large part of humic acid takes and active part in the liver metabolism makes sense for the further study of the influence on hepatitis." Conclusion: Humic acid has a great future for use in medicine and veterinary sciences due to high potential of biological activity, antitoxin properties of humic acid, protective effect in cases of disturbance of physiological functions and simulative effect on the mechanism of resistance.

Medical Aspects and Applications of Humic Substances Regarding the Antiviral Activity of Humic Substance

By Prof. Dr. Renate Klocking & Dr. rer. nat. Bjorn Helbig, Institute for Antiviral Chemotherapy, Friedrich Schiller University, Jena, Germany. 25 Sept.2013

Research indicates that Humic Acids functions both prophylactically as well as therapeutically in the treatment of viral diseases.

Humic Acid is first a preventative, because it interferes with a virus' ability to attach to a host cell, penetrate the host cell, and reproduce itself. Scientific studies have demonstrated that if a host cell is penetrated before the introduction of the Humic Acid, the viral reproductive process within the host cell is not halted.

HOWEVER, if one has latently infected cells (i.e. those with chronic viral infections) and Humic Acid is present, once the host cell releases the new viruses into the bloodstream the Humic Acid helps prevent the new generation(s) of viruses from attaching to the cell wall, hijacking the DNA or RNA and reproducing, effectively lowering the body's viral load over time and hence its therapeutic function for active viral infections. Humic Acid may work for most, if not all, viral infections. Other studies are currently on going throughout the world.

Protocol for taking humic acid:

- normal adult prophylactic use: one (1) capsule per day, every day
- normal child prophylactic use: one-half (1/2) capsule per day every day
- adult prophylactic use when at risk (i.e., during flu season): two (2) capsules, one in the morning and one in the evening, then resume normal prophylactic dose after the risk has passed.
- adult therapeutic use if in the midst of a cold, flu, or other non-life threatening viral illness: three (3) capsules per day, one each in the morning, noon, and at bedtime, for 2-3 days or until symptoms subside, then adjust dose to two (2) capsules per day (one each in the morning, and evening).
- adult therapeutic does for Hepatitis A, B, C: one (1) capsule three times a day for 4-6 weeks. Thereafter, take one (1) capsule twice daily to help the body's immune system. Drink lots of clean, purified electrolyte water during the day.
- adult therapeutic use for Herpes (oral/genital, Epstein-Barr, Shingles and other herpes viruses): two (2) capsules three times a day while the outbreak persists. Thereafter, take one (1) capsule twice daily to help the body's immune system.
- normal pet prophylactic use (dogs & cats): one-half (1/2) capsule per day for small pets; one (1) capsule per day for large pets.

Frequently Asked Questions about Humic Acid

What is Humic acid?
- Humic acid has been discovered to be a significant miracle of nature. A part of the humate structure of enriched composting soil, it has been the subject of extensive scientific research, the body's ability to maintain over all health.

How can Humic acid help the body's immune system combat different illnesses?
- All animal viruses must bind to host cells in order to reproduce. Humic acid has been shown in numerous vitro studies to block this fusion process (including AIDS, Herpes, Influenza and hemorrhagic fever). The immune system then eliminates these viruses.

Is it safe?
- Humic acid has undergone extensive in vivo testing at levels 50-100 times higher than would be used in practice, with no detectable signs of toxicity.

Can I take Humic acid with other medication?
- As far as it is known, humic acid has no drug interactions and no side effects.

How long do I need to take Humic Acid?
- The suggested use of humic acid as a dietary supplement is similar to taking a multivitamin. Even in the absence of illness, it is strongly recommended taking 1-2 tablets a day.

How long until I begin to see results?
- Humic acid is completely water-soluble and it enters the body within minutes of being taken in table from. It then begins acting immediately to aid the body's ability to maintain its overall health.

Can I give this to my pets?

- Yes. Humic acid is an excellent prevention for parvovirus, a highly contagious disease for dogs, West Nile virus in other pets and livestock animals.

Testimonials

Viral Immunity with Humic Acid for Humans:

Influenza

"Recently I came down with a very bad case of influenza. Normally this leads to severe respiratory distress. I was given humic acid to take every six hours. Within forty-eight hours, all my symptoms were gone. I am very grateful for this product and I will continue to keep humic acid in my house for myself and family members."

Meg C., Santa Fe, NM

Hepatitis C

"A year ago I was diagnosed with hepatitis C. A friend suggested I start taking humic acid. I was tested again six weeks later and the results were negative. the doctors could not believe that the hepatitis C was gone. Thank you, thank you."

Gary D., Dallas, TX

AIDS/HIV

"I stared recommending humic acid for my HIV+ patients and I am amazed how fast their viral loads are reduced. I plan to use this product with my other patients that are diagnosed with Hepatitis, Epstein-Barr and other various viral infections."

Dr. Hugo Garza, Guadalajara, Mexico

Herpes

"For the last fifteen years I have lived with genital herpes. About once a month I would expect and outbreak. The medication I was taking was not helping. I began taking humic acid at the suggested dosage and the infection cleared up in a few days. I take a daily dose of one table, and I have not had a recurrence."

Denise Z., Cleveland, OH

For General Health

"I have been taking humic acid for six months, once a day. I am 87 years young and have not had a cold nor the flue, even though my doctor recommended me getting the flu shot."

Al P., Orlando, FL

Cold sores

"I used to get cold sores and fever blisters at least once a month. I was then introduced and stared taking humic acid. I have been on the product for over three months and have not had any outbreaks. I am very grateful for humic acid."

Larry S., Orlando, FL

West Nile Virus

"I live in the southwest and because I am constantly working outside on my ranch, my exposure rate to the West Nile virus is extremely high. To prevent getting this virus my family and myself take humic acid daily. I am also giving humic acid to my horses to help prevent them from getting the virus. I would highly recommend to everyone to take humic acid."

Lazaro G., Taos, NM

Hepatitis C

"One of my clients who was diagnosed with Hepatitis C, started taking humic acid four weeks ago. He recently had his viral load tested and the results came back undetectable. I am very impressed with this product and plan to recommend humic acid to all my clients for either preventing and/or benefiting various viral conditions."

Dr. Dennis Kramer, Santa Fe, NM

Viral Immunity with Humic Acid for Animals:

"I recently had a three pound Pom pick up a virus and the medication from the vet wasn't working. A friend suggested giving her humic acid.

I opened the capsule and sprinkled it on her food. I continued doing this for a few days and each day my pup continued to improve. I really believe the humic acid helped to save my Sweetie's life."

Tom D., Baltimore, MD

"I love cats and there was a litter of kittens born on my farm to a family of 'barn' cats. As soon as they were weaned, the kittens were given a home, except one. We kept that one, the 'runt' of the litter. In her daily diet we included humic acid. Several months later all the kittens from the litter tested positive for Feline Leukemia Virus (FeLV). We continued to give our kitten humic acid. Sadly the other kittens died. Our Tiffy, from that same litter, is now almost 8 years old and still acts like a kitten."

Sally G., Portland, OR

"One of my race horses developed virus symptoms and was to be scratched from the racing program scheduled the following day. I gave some humic acid to the animal and he improved sufficiently enough to enter the race. He hit the board first, second, and third."

Patrick L., Toronto, ON

"I service large animals in an eight-county area. This area of the country has large feedlots containing as many as 100,000 head of cattle. This also is horse country, the workers using horses to work with the cattle. West Nile Virus has been a problem here for the last three years. Even animals with vaccinations for the disease have been diagnosed with West Nile. I find that humic acid is an excellent antiviral to give to those affected. Generally within 24 to 36 hours, symptoms of the disease abated. To the extreme, I have had horses that were down and vision impaired by the brain swelling and brought them back with humic acid. In my opinion, humic acid is as or more effective then antibiotics that are recommended."

Tom S., DMV, Guymon, OK

Resource Directory

Humic acid is available in a variety of forms. However, not every form is formulated with viral fusion inhibitors. Below is the source I recommend:

Humisol   **www.healthbesttoday.com**   **866-777-5050**

About The Author

Dr. Howard Peiper is a Doctor of Naturopathic Medicine. In 1972, he received his degree in Naturopathy. After a decade in private practice, Dr. Peiper became a successful consultant, speaker and writer.

Throughout the years, his cutting-edge articles appeared in numerous medical journals and magazines. He also serves on the medical advisory board for several nutritional companies.

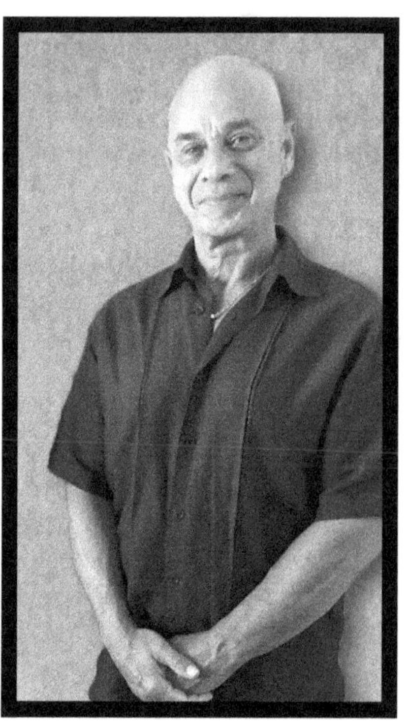

Dr. Peiper has written several bestselling titles, including: The A.D.D. and A.D.H.D. Diet, The secrets to Staying Young and New Hope for Serious Diseases. He is a frequent guest speaker on radio and television programs. He even hosted his own shows, including the award-winning television shot "Partners in Healing."

Notes

Notes

Notes

Notes

* 9 7 9 8 6 9 2 5 6 8 9 9 1 *